C000093637

CHRONIC NECK PAIN

The Essential Guide to Finding Neck Pain Relief

Copyright © 2018 by Veritas Health, LLC
ISBN: 978-0-9965175-2-2
Edited by Grant Cooper, MD

This book is not intended as a substitute for the medical advice of physicians. The reader
should regularly consult a physician in matters relating to his/her health and particularly with
respect to any symptoms that may require diagnosis or medical attention.

All rights reserved. No part of this publication may be reproduced, distributed, or transmitted
in any form or by any means, including photocopying, recording, or other electronic or
mechanical methods, without the prior written permission of Veritas Health, LLC, except in
the case of brief quotations embodied in critical reviews and certain other noncommercial uses
permitted by copyright law. For permission requests, write to Veritas Health, LLC, addressed
"Attention: Legal," at the address below.

Veritas Health
520 Lake Cook Road, Suite 350
Deerfield, IL 60015
VeritasHealth.com
Spine-health.com
Arthritis-health.com
Sports-health.com
Pain-health.com

First Edition, 2018

TABLE OF CONTENTS

For my wife and best friend, Ana, and our children, Mila, Lara, and Luka.

For my colleagues, friends, and family at Princeton Spine and Joint Center.

And for my patients, who inspire me as much as I strive to honor them.

Finally, for my parents, who set me on this path.

—Grant Cooper, MD

ABOUT THIS BOOK

Neck pain that persists for weeks or months is frustrating, especially when the pain goes beyond the typical stiff neck or dull ache. For some people, neck pain can become sharp, with symptoms of shock-like pain, pins-and-needles tingling, weakness, and/or numbness radiating down the shoulder, arm, and/or hand. In the worst cases, pain can become so bad that it interferes with daily activities and quality of life.

The goals of this book are to help you better understand your condition and symptoms, as well as give you information about how to get an accurate diagnosis and consider your treatment options. This book can also be kept as a handy reference, or given to a loved one who wants to better understand what you're going through.

The information in this book has been peer-reviewed and can also be found in different formats in doctor-authored, peer-reviewed articles and videos published on Spine-health.com. Both this book and the website have been developed according to a rigorous and unbiased medical review process.

For more detailed information on the many medical conditions and procedures described in this book, visit Spine-health.com.

ABOUT VERITAS HEALTH

Since 1999 Veritas Health, LLC has provided unbiased, comprehensive, and trusted content to millions of people, empowering them to make informed decisions regarding their health. With over 20 million pageviews each month, the Veritas Health platform comprising of Spine-health.com, Arthritis-health.com, Sports-health.com, and Pain-health.com, provides comprehensive information on back pain, arthritis, sports injuries, and chronic pain conditions. For more information visit Veritashealth.com.

1.

THE NECK
AND WHAT CAN GO WRONG

Necks are true marvels of biomechanical engineering. All day, every day, your neck holds up your head, which weighs a little more than a bowling ball. All of the head's turns and tilts are accomplished so seamlessly that most of us don't even think about the neck—until it hurts.

So how does the neck become painful? Let's review the basics of neck anatomy and what can cause discomfort.

THE FORM AND FUNCTION OF THE NECK

The neck runs from the base of the skull down to the top of the chest. Some of the neck's important functions include enabling head movements and facilitating the flow of blood and electrical signals between the brain and the rest of the body.

The spinal region that runs through the neck is called the cervical spine, which is comprised of:

- **VERTEBRAE.** These bones are stacked vertically to provide both support and flexibility for the neck and head, forming the spinal column that protects the spinal cord within.

- **INTERVERTEBRAL DISCS.** Between adjacent vertebrae is an intervertebral disc that cushions the bones so they don't grind against each other while the neck moves.

- **NERVE ROOTS.** At each spinal level, two nerve roots (one on each side) branch off from the spinal cord and go through small openings in the vertebrae to carry signals that control movement and feeling in different parts of the body.

The neck's cervical spine is held together and moved by soft tissues such as muscles, tendons, and ligaments. By far the most common type of neck pain is when one or more of these soft tissues become overextended and/or slightly torn. Fortunately, these strains and sprains usually go away on their own within a week or two.

If neck pain instead stems from a problem with a vertebra, disc, joint, or nerve root, the symptoms can last much longer and require more extensive treatment.

CERVICAL VERTEBRAE AND FACET JOINT PAIN

There are seven cervical vertebrae, numbered C1 through C7. The C1 vertebra at the top of the cervical spine is the smallest. The vertebrae get progressively bigger going down the spine. C7 is the biggest cervical vertebra so it can support C6 above it, and so on.

The C1 and C2 vertebrae both have atypical shapes due to their unique roles at the top of the cervical spine. C1, called the atlas, is connected to the skull and allows about 50% of the head's forward/backward range of motion. C2, called the axis, is connected beneath C1 and above C3, and allows about 50% of the neck's rotation.

The rest of the neck's rotation, forward, and backward movements are distributed amongst the vertebrae C3 through C7, which all share these basic characteristics:

- **VERTEBRAL BODY.** The thick cylindrical front of each vertebral bone is called the vertebral body, which handles most of the load and stress placed on the spine. At each vertebral level, a soft but sturdy disc sits between the vertebral bodies that are stacked on top of each other.

- **VERTEBRAL ARCH.** Comprised of two pedicles and two laminae, the vertebral arch is the bony protection that forms the backside of the spinal canal where the spinal cord runs within the vertebra.

- **FACET JOINTS.** A paired set of facet joints are located toward the back of each vertebra where the pedicle and lamina connect. Facet joints are the only true synovial joints within

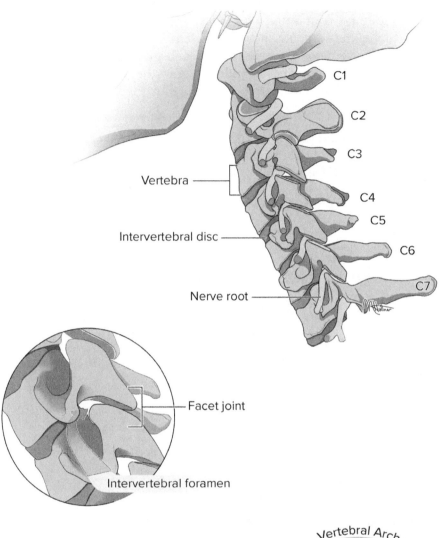

C1
C2
C3
Vertebra
C4
C5
Intervertebral disc
C6
Nerve root
C7

Facet joint

Intervertebral foramen

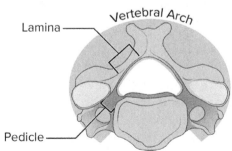

Lamina

Vertebral Arch

Pedicle

Superior view of C4

the spine, containing a joint capsule and lined with cartilage to facilitate smooth movements. These joints are small and the movements are restricted at each spinal level, but these limited movements can add up to give the cervical spine significant amounts of rotation, forward/backward, and side-to-side movements.

When neck pain lasts for more than a few weeks, a common cause is a problem in the facet joint, such as a tear in the cartilage or degeneration of the joint.

CERVICAL DISCS AND DISCOGENIC PAIN

There are six intervertebral discs in the cervical spine. Each disc includes:

- **ANNULUS FIBROSUS.** This tough outer layer is made out of collagen fibers, which give the disc its sturdiness and protect the softer inner layer.

- **NUCLEUS PULPOSUS.** This jelly-like interior is a loose, fibrous network suspended in mucoprotein gel and sealed within the annulus fibrosus.

Discogenic pain is pain that comes from the disc itself, which can occur if there is a tear in the disc due to trauma or degeneration.

NERVE ROOTS AND RELATED PAIN

There are 8 pairs of spinal nerve roots in the cervical spine. These cervical nerve roots are named C1 through C8. Most cervical nerve roots are named after the vertebra beneath it, but the C8 nerve root runs below the C7 vertebra and above the T1 vertebra.

On both sides of a vertebra, there is a small hole or opening (called a foramen, which is formed by the bottom of the vertebra above and the top of the vertebra below) where the nerve root travels through as it branches from the spinal cord and carries signals to a specific region of the body. Nerve roots in the neck feed into nerves that run down into the shoulder, arm, hand, and/or fingers.

If a nerve root becomes irritated, such as from a herniated disc or bone spur rubbing against it, cervical radicular pain and/or cervical radiculopathy can occur. Cervical radicular pain is associated with tingling, aching, electrical-like sensations that may travel part or all of the way down the nerve and be felt in faraway body regions such as the arm or fingers—but without any change in neurological function (sensation, reflexes and/or weakness). Cervical radiculopathy may also involve tingling, aching, and electrical-like sensations but additionally must cause a change in neurological function (sensation, reflexes and/or weakness). So you can have radicular pain without having a radiculopathy, but usually not have a radiculopathy without some form of radicular pain.

While many medical professionals refer to symptomatic nerve roots as being pinched or impinged, a true mechanical impingement of a nerve root is rare. It is the inflammation of the nerve root that causes radicular pain, while cervical radiculopathy must be associated with a change in neurological function.

MUSCLES AND MYOFASCIAL PAIN

Numerous muscles help support and move the cervical spine. If one or more of these muscles develops pain that persists or recurs over a period of several months, it is most likely due to an underlying problem in the cervical spine. For example, a degenerating cervical disc can cause inflammation, and a nearby muscle could start spasming and become painful in response. While the muscle may be painful, the underlying cause is the degenerating disc. In a sense, the muscle spasms as a way of "guarding" or "protecting" the underlying disc. Ironically, this spasm is often more painful than the underlying spinal problem.

In some cases, however, a neck muscle can become chronically painful without an identifiable underlying cause in the cervical spine. While this tends to be much less common, chronic neck pain stemming from one or more muscles is known as cervical myofascial pain syndrome.

For more information, read *Cervical Spine Anatomy and Neck Pain*: spine-health.com/ebook/cnp/link1

2.

COMMON NECK PAIN SYMPTOMS

Neck pain and associated symptoms can take many forms, depending on what's causing the pain, the extent of the damage, and your own body's way of detecting pain.

Symptoms most commonly associated with neck pain include one or more of the following:

- **STIFF NECK.** Moving the head becomes difficult due to pain, especially when attempting to turn the head to the side.

- **SHARP PAIN.** Localized in one spot, this pain can feel like it's stinging or stabbing. When experienced in the neck, sharp pain is usually, though not always, in the lower levels.

- **GENERAL SORENESS.** This pain feels tender or achy. It usually covers a bigger region rather than one small spot.

- **CERVICAL RADICULAR PAIN.** When a nerve root in the neck becomes inflamed and painful but neurological deficits are absent, it is called radicular pain. Cervical radicular pain is associated with tingling, aching, electrical-like sensations that may travel part or all of the way down the nerve and be felt in faraway body regions such as the arm or fingers—but without any change in neurological function (sensation, reflexes and/ or weakness). This pain may feel burning or shock-like, and it can radiate down into the shoulder, arm, and/or hand. Radicular pain is typically only on one side of the body, but it can be felt on both sides in some cases. It may come and go.

- **CERVICAL RADICULOPATHY.** When a nerve in the neck becomes damaged and causes a change in neurological function, it is called cervical radiculopathy. Cervical radiculopathy may also involve tingling, aching, and electrical like sensations but additionally must cause a change in neurological function (sensation, reflexes and/or weakness). So, you can have cervical radicular pain without having a radiculopathy, but usually not have a radiculopathy without some form of radicular pain. Cervical radiculopathy tends to be on only one side of the body or the other, typically is constant, and might be exacerbated by certain neck movements or positions. If pain, weakness, and/or numbness go into the hands, it could cause difficulty with gripping or lifting objects.

- **HEADACHES.** An aggravation in the neck can also affect muscles and/or nerves connected to the head. This pain could be at the base of the skull or up the sides of the head or even the scalp. Sometimes people develop what is termed a cervicogenic headache in which pain in the head (often localized to behind the eye or the back of the head) is referred directly from the cervical spine. Some instances of cervicogenic headache occur in the absence of actual neck pain. Cervicogenic headaches can be unilateral (on one side) or bilateral (on both sides).

If neck pain symptoms become severe enough, they can start interfering with daily activities. Some examples could include difficulty with driving, getting dressed, typing, or even sleeping.

SYMPTOMS BY SPINAL NERVE LOCATION

Each spinal nerve exiting the spinal cord goes to a different part of the body. Depending on which spinal nerve is inflamed will determine which area of the body experiences symptoms. Common examples in the cervical spine include the following:

- C5 nerve impingement can cause weakness in the shoulder and/or biceps. In addition, pain, tingling and numbness may radiate into the upper arm and thumb.

- C6 nerve impingement can lead to weakness in the biceps and wrist. In addition, pain, tingling, and numbness can radiate through the arm to the second digit.

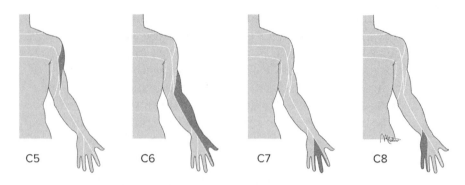

C5   C6   C7   C8

These images only show the arms as viewed from the front. For example, C7 also powers the triceps muscle at the back of the arm, which is not shown.

- C7 nerve impingement can cause weakness in the back of the upper arm (triceps), and pain can radiate down the arm and into the middle finger.

- C8 nerve impingement can result in handgrip weakness, along with numbness and tingling pain that radiates down the arm to the little finger.

While much less common, it is possible for more than one spinal nerve to be inflamed at the same time.

ONSET OF NECK PAIN SYMPTOMS

Neck pain typically begins in one of the following ways:

- **SUDDENLY.** Sometimes neck pain develops immediately with or without an obvious reason. Perhaps it starts right after a fall, or maybe it appears out of the blue one evening while relaxing at home.

- **GRADUALLY.** Neck pain might begin as a mild nuisance, go away, and then keep coming back. For example, you might notice a minor neck pain at the end of each work day, and over time that pain might slowly start earlier in the day, get worse, and possibly stop going away completely.

- **DELAYED.** Neck pain doesn't always start immediately following damage to it. Sometimes the pain can start hours, days, weeks or longer after an accident has happened. A common example is when the neck sustains a whiplash injury in a car accident.

Chronic neck pain can vary in intensity over time, with the pain subsiding during some periods before flaring up and becoming more intense at other times. In other cases, chronic neck pain can be constant, such as a deep, achy throb that seemingly never goes away and/or always intensifies during certain movements.

For more information, read *Neck Pain Symptoms*:
spine-health.com/ebook/cnp/link2

3.

COMMON CAUSES OF CHRONIC NECK PAIN

Back in Chapter 1, we looked at some general ways the neck can become painful. Now let's explore more specifically the common causes of chronic neck pain.

SPINAL DEGENERATION

Whether from natural wear and tear over time, genetic predisposition, injury, or some combination thereof, spinal degeneration can lead to painful problems within the neck.

Cervical spondylosis is an umbrella term for the spinal degeneration and associated problems that can occur when the cervical spine's discs and spinal joints start to wear down and become inflamed. Disc degeneration may begin first, then result in more stress on the facet joints and uncovertebral joints, which can eventually start to grow osteophytes (bone spurs) as the body tries to maintain spinal stability.

Some specific conditions that can cause neck pain include:

- **CERVICAL DEGENERATIVE DISC DISEASE.** As the intervertebral discs lose hydration, they begin to flatten so their ability to cushion adjacent vertebral bones decreases and pain may occur. For example, small nerves in the disc's outer layer (annulus fibrosus) could become irritated, or inflammatory proteins from the inner layer (nucleus pulposus) could leak outward onto these same nerves and cause pain.

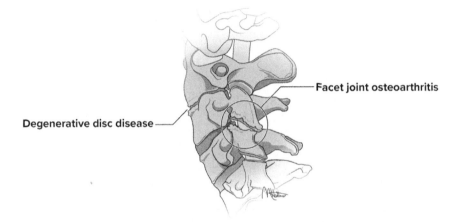

Facet joint osteoarthritis

Degenerative disc disease

- **CERVICAL FACET JOINT OSTEOARTHRITIS.** When the protective cartilage within a facet joint starts to wear down and no longer supports smooth movements between the vertebral bones, inflammation occurs and bone spurs may grow in an effort to stabilize the swollen, arthritic joint. As the osteoarthritis progresses, the facet joint enlarges and may become painful and possibly press against or irritate a nearby nerve root. Cervical facet joint osteoarthritis is one of the most common causes of chronic neck pain.

- **CERVICAL HERNIATED DISC.** When part or all of the disc's protective outer layer (annulus fibrosus) tears, some of the central nucleus pulposus may leak into the tear and cause inflammation and pain. If the disc bulges but the nucleus pulposus remains inside the annulus, it is referred to as a contained disc herniation. If the nucleus pulposus leaks outside the annulus, it is an uncontained disc herniation and may cause irritation in nearby structures, such as a nerve root.

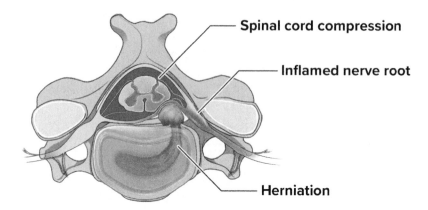

- **CERVICAL FORAMINAL STENOSIS.** When the foramen (bony hole where the nerve root exits the spinal canal) narrows— such as from a bone spur or a herniated disc —the nerve root has less space and may become compressed and/or inflamed.

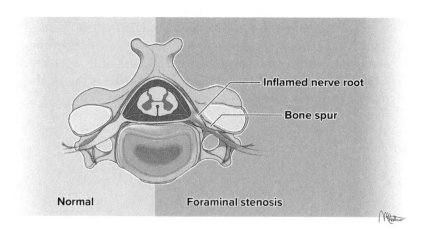

- **CERVICAL SPINAL STENOSIS.** This condition occurs when the spinal canal narrows (stenosis) and symptoms of spinal cord compression may be exhibited (myelopathic symptoms), which are usually bilateral, such as tingling and/or pain in both arms and possibly also legs. Various problems can cause the spinal canal to narrow, such as bone spurs, thickening ligaments, degenerating discs, and others. When myelopathic symptoms also cause a loss of strength, sensation, reflexes, or bowel and/or bladder control, then the condition is called a myelopathy.

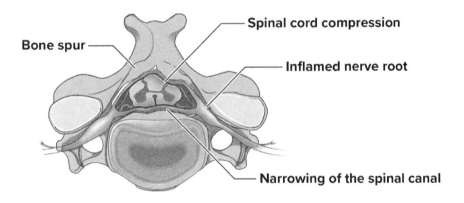

Spinal cord compression

Bone spur

Inflamed nerve root

Narrowing of the spinal canal

POOR POSTURE

Good neck posture involves keeping the head in a neutral position with the ears directly above the shoulders. Whenever you deviate from this positioning for long periods of time, the cervical spine's discs, joints, muscles, and other soft tissues must do more work and undergo more stress. The muscles and soft tissues become overstretched and/or tightened, which can become painful.

In today's world, it's common for people who work long hours hunched over a computer to develop neck pain. Other possible ways that poor posture can lead to neck pain include manual labor jobs that require lots of heavy lifting, or hobbies that involve holding the head at odd angles, such as tending to a large garden.

Neck pain from poor posture may be only temporary, but it can become chronic if the poor posture is regularly repeated or if it exacerbates other conditions, such as cervical degenerative disc disease or cervical facet joint osteoarthritis.

TRAUMATIC INJURY

A collision or accident may cause damage to the discs, joints, muscles, ligaments, bones, and/or other tissues in the neck. Some common examples include:

- **Auto accident**

- **Bike accident**

- **Sports collision, such as in football or hockey**

- **Slip on ice or wet floor**

- **Fall from height, such as down steps or a ladder**

While the acute injury from a collision or accident typically heals and the pain goes away, sometimes neck pain lingers and becomes chronic even after the injury has healed. There are various theories as to why chronic neck pain can last after an injury has healed. It could be due to permanent disc or facet joint dysfunction and inflammation, an acceleration of preexisting spinal degeneration, or psychosocial factors related to mental health and overall wellbeing, among other possibilities.

The neck pain from an accident may not occur right away. For example, pain from an automobile whiplash injury may take a day, weeks or much longer before occurring. In other cases, neck pain from a traumatic injury may resolve but then return several years later and become chronic.

**Watch our video to understand more about whiplash:
spine-health.com/ebook/cnp/link13**

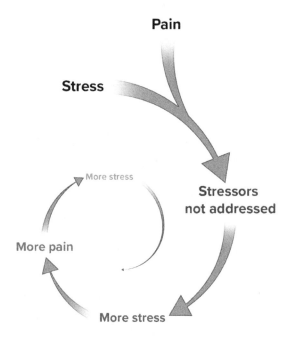

Current research indicates that chronic neck and back pain is more common in people who have anxiety, depression, or other mental health issues. The reason for this is still not clear, but it could be related to various types of ongoing stress, such as social isolation and financial struggles. Another possibility is that people who are prone to anxiety and/or depression might perceive pain differently than other people.

Many people with neck pain (and other sorts of pain) may notice an increase in pain when undergoing a particularly stressful period in their life. This is normal. When you are under stress, it is harder to cope with pain. This is similar to a lack of sleep. If you don't get a good night's sleep, your pain may feel worse because you are less able to cope with it. Not realizing or acknowledging this association between stress and pain may ironically make the pain worse.

For more information, read *Neck Pain Causes*:
spine-health.com/ebook/cnp/link3

4.

WHEN NECK PAIN REQUIRES A VISIT TO THE DOCTOR

Most people will experience neck pain at some point in their lives. So how can you tell the difference between neck pain that will go away on its own and neck pain that requires a visit to the doctor? Here are some tips.

WHEN TO MAKE AN APPOINTMENT

Typically, you should visit a doctor if one or more of the following is true about your neck pain:

- **IT CONTINUES TO INTERFERE WITH DAILY ACTIVITIES.** Does your neck pain interfere with routine tasks, such as dressing, concentrating, or sleeping? If giving your neck a rest and/or trying an over-the-counter pain reliever does not provide enough relief after a couple days, visit a doctor.

- **IT LASTS MORE THAN A COUPLE WEEKS.** If the pain is not noticeably better after a couple of weeks, it could be a sign that the problem will linger unless medical attention is sought.

- **IT RADIATES INTO THE ARM.** Any pain or tingling that radiates into the shoulders or arms should be examined by a doctor. If numbness and/or weakness are experienced anywhere in the shoulder, arm, hand, and/or fingers, seek immediate medical attention.

When neck pain symptoms are limited to the neck and seem to be getting better on their own, there is usually no need to visit the doctor. However, if you experience acute neck pain that goes away on its own but continues to return, you should visit the doctor.

WHEN NECK PAIN SYMPTOMS NEED IMMEDIATE ATTENTION

Sometimes neck pain accompanies a more serious underlying condition, such as a spinal cord injury, cancer, HIV, meningitis, or other conditions. Immediately seek medical attention if you experience neck pain with any of the following:

- **Fever or chills**

- **Radiating pain in both arms and/or legs**

- **Numbness, tingling, or weakness in both arms and/or legs**

- **Problems with balance or coordination**

- **Loss of bowel or bladder control**

- **Unintended weight loss**

When severe neck pain results from major trauma, such as a car accident or falling down steps, it should be treated as a medical emergency.

**For more information, read *When Is a Stiff Neck Serious*:
spine-health.com/ebook/cnp/link4**

5.

NECK PAIN DIAGNOSIS

When your neck hurts, it's natural to want to know why. Finding the underlying cause of neck pain can help determine an effective course of treatment.

In order to diagnose the cause of neck pain, a doctor will take your medical history and perform a physical examination. If more information is needed to further narrow down the cause, advanced diagnostics may also be requested.

STEP 1: REVIEW YOUR MEDICAL HISTORY

In addition to learning about your medical past, such as prior surgeries or known chronic conditions, the doctor will ask about:

- **NECK PAIN SYMPTOMS.** When did you first notice the symptoms? Does the pain feel sharp, dull, or something else? Do the symptoms worsen or improve during certain activities?

- **LIFESTYLE.** How do you spend a typical day? What type of work or hobbies do you do? What does your workstation look like? Are you regularly performing physically strenuous tasks or perhaps sitting a lot?

- **PRIOR INJURIES.** Do you recall something recent that might have triggered the neck pain, such as a bike accident or lifting something heavy? How about an event from further back in time, such as an old sports injury or a scary fall that has stuck in your mind?

As the doctor learns more about your symptoms, habits, and medical past, the line of questioning may alter depending on which conditions can and cannot be ruled out.

For example, how you spend a typical day could provide clues about what's aggravating your neck. If your neck pain is bad when you wake up but gets better as the day goes on, perhaps adjusting your sleep position or getting a different pillow will do the trick. If your neck pain tends to be worse at the end of the work day, maybe adjusting your workstation to become more ergonomic could provide relief.

STEP 2: PHYSICAL EXAMINATION

After reviewing your medical history and symptoms, the doctor narrows the list of possible causes for your neck pain. To further investigate, a physical exam of your neck is performed and typically includes:

- **OBSERVATION.** The neck is inspected for any lesions, abnormalities, or poor posture (particularly as regards to the head, neck, and shoulders).

- **PALPATION.** The neck's soft tissues are carefully pushed and felt for any indications of muscle spasms, tightness, or tenderness.

- **RANGE OF MOTION TEST.** The head is tilted forward and backward, side to side, and rotated to see if any range of motion has been lost, or if certain movements exacerbate pain.

- **REFLEXES.** A rubber hammer can examine reflexes in the biceps, triceps, and forearm. If the reflexes are decreased or absent, nerves in the neck may not be sending signals as intended.

- **STRENGTH.** By having you apply different types of pressure or squeezing, pushing and pulling, your doctor will check for obvious signs of weakness in the shoulders, arms, and hands.

- **SENSATION.** Your doctor will check your arms and hands with light touch or perhaps a cotton tip for your ability to perceive sensation equally and normally on both sides.

- **PAINFUL MOVEMENTS.** Your doctor might perform Spurling's test, which involves having you extend and rotate your head to the symptomatic side. He or she then gently pushes down on your head to see if that reproduces (or temporarily worsens) your symptoms.

POSSIBLE STEP 3: ADVANCED DIAGNOSTICS

When the patient history and physical examination do not provide enough information for the doctor to formulate a treatment plan, diagnostic imaging may be considered. It is important to remember that any imaging study alone—MRI, CT, or x-ray—does not tell what is causing your pain. However, the combination of your history, physical examination, and imaging (if needed) are the most common ways to narrow down the diagnosis.

Some common diagnostic imaging studies that your doctor may order include:

- **MRI SCAN.** A magnetic resonance imaging (MRI) scan uses a strong magnet and radio waves to detect variations in anatomical structures. This information is utilized to create a series of detailed cross-sections of the soft tissues and bones. Compared to an x-ray or CT scan, an MRI gives a superior view of the soft tissues, such as nerves and discs, which is why it is the most common imaging performed when trying to diagnose chronic neck pain.

- **CT SCAN WITH MYELOGRAM.** A computerized tomography (CT) scan takes multiple x-rays of the body region being studied, which in this case is the cervical spine. A computer then generates a series of images to show the bones in much greater detail than a traditional x-ray or MRI. A myelogram may be performed ahead of time with a contrast dye injected into the sac surrounding the nerve roots to help better visualize them on the CT scan.

Other diagnostic tests that might be considered include fluoroscopically-guided, contrast-enhanced injections in or around various structures (such as to verify that a facet joint or spinal nerve is the source of pain), electrodiagnostic testing (for nerve and muscle function), somatosensory evoked potentials (for spinal cord issues), blood tests, and others.

NECK PAIN DIAGNOSIS MAY BE ELUSIVE

Despite today's modern technologies, the specific source of chronic neck pain is not always possible to diagnose. For example, a person's MRI might show significant degeneration at one part of the cervical spine, but the symptoms might feel as though they are coming from a completely different part of the spine.

While it can be especially frustrating to have chronic neck pain without being able to diagnose the exact cause, there is a silver lining here. When neck pain remains difficult to diagnose, it is unlikely to be due to a dangerous underlying condition. Serious or life-threatening causes of neck pain are typically a clear-cut diagnosis.

It should be noted that the vast majority of cases of chronic neck pain can be diagnosed.

**For more information, read *Diagnosing Neck Pain*:
spine-health.com/ebook/cnp/link5**

6.

SELF-CARE TREATMENT OPTIONS

Sometimes neck pain can be managed on your own. Depending on your specific symptoms, one or more of the treatments discussed in this chapter may work for you.

SHORT PERIODS OF REST

Whenever you have a bad flare-up of neck pain, it's a good idea to go easy and avoid strenuous activities that could potentially worsen the pain. Trying to soldier on despite bad pain is likely to just make it last longer and hurt worse.

While rest is sometimes necessary for a painful neck, too much rest can also be bad. When the neck is immobilized or forced to rest for too long, such as for more than a few days, neck muscles can weaken and become more susceptible to painful muscle spasms.

COLD THERAPY

Within the first 24 to 48 hours of neck pain starting or worsening, applying ice or cold packs to the neck can help. Ice or cold packs temporarily close small blood vessels and reduce swelling. That is why ice therapy is most effective when used early to prevent the swelling from becoming worse, as opposed to waiting until the swelling has already reached its maximum potential.

Cold therapy can be applied to the neck for about 10 to 20 minutes at a time, with at least a 2-hour break in between sessions. Ice should always be placed within a cloth of some type to avoid direct contact with the skin. Otherwise, the skin tissue could become damaged if it's exposed to too much cold.

HEAT THERAPY

For ongoing chronic neck pain, many people find significant relief from heat therapy. Applying heat to the neck can help reduce pain by relaxing painful muscles and distracting the brain's pain receptors. Heat may also promote healing by increasing blood flow that brings nutrients to the injured area.

There are many types of heat therapy, and you might want to try different ones before deciding which works best. Some people prefer wet heat, such as taking a warm bath or shower, soaking in a hot tub, or applying a towel that has soaked in hot water. Dry heat options could include microwavable heat packs, electric heating pads, or chemical heat packs.

Heat therapy is best used for 15 or 20 minutes per treatment, no more than one treatment every 2 hours. When applying a heat pack, include a layer between the heat source and your skin to avoid a burn. Also, when using a heating pad, take care to avoid falling asleep, which could result in excessive heat exposure and skin damage—even if the heat is set to low.

ACTIVE LIFESTYLE

The neck craves movement, which is necessary to keep joints limber and nutrients flowing to bones and soft tissues. When you live a sedentary lifestyle, muscles weaken, joints stiffen, and the heart pumps blood less efficiently. Regularly failing to get enough movement can exacerbate neck pain.

Instead, make a plan to stay active throughout the day. If you watch TV shows, try to get up and move during commercial breaks. If your job mostly involves sitting at a desk, schedule short breaks every 30 or 60 minutes when possible. Have a long commute? Consider whether the warmer months offer opportunities to get off the train one stop early, bike to work, or perhaps park a good walking distance from the office.

ACTIVITY MODIFICATION

While it is important to stay active for spine health, certain activities may cause problems for some people. For example, if twisting the head to the side while swimming freestyle causes you pain, perhaps consider swimming that stroke less often or sticking to strokes that don't require twisting the neck in that manner. Another option if you like freestyle but it causes pain is to use a snorkel while you swim to eliminate the breathing side-to-side.

OVER-THE-COUNTER MEDICATIONS

Sometimes an over-the-counter medication can provide adequate relief for neck pain. Some examples include acetaminophen (e.g. Tylenol) or non-steroidal anti-inflammatory drugs, also called NSAIDs (e.g. Advil, Aleve, Motrin).

Just because a medication is readily available over-the-counter doesn't mean it's without risks. Carefully read drug labels and follow directions before usage. Also, if you take more than one medication, pay attention to active ingredients listed in the drug label to avoid an accidental overdose. For instance, acetaminophen can be found in more than just pain medicines, such as cold medicines, allergy medicines, and others.

PRACTICE GOOD POSTURE AND ERGONOMICS

Tilting the head forward increases pressure on the cervical spine. When the head is held forward for too long, such as while hunched over a computer or staring down at a smartphone, the neck may eventually become painful.

Using good posture keeps the spine better aligned and less stressed. Simple changes can be made, such as altering a workstation to ensure that your chair, monitor, and keyboard are positioned in ways to keep the body, head, and neck more aligned in a natural position; or learning to sleep on the back (instead of the stomach or side) with an ergonomically friendly pillow and mattress. Using a headset if you spend a lot of time on the telephone can likewise be helpful.

HEALTHY EATING

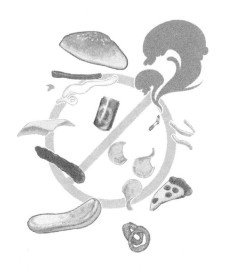 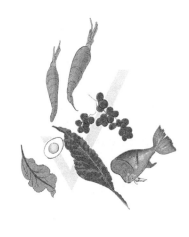

What you eat plays an important role in how you feel, both physically and emotionally. Eating a well-balanced, nutritious diet will help give you the energy to follow your treatment plan for neck pain, as well as boost your mood.

Current research suggests that limiting high-inflammation foods may reduce pain in the body. Try to limit the intake of processed foods, junk foods, soda, and refined grains (such as white bread). Instead, focus on getting plenty of fruits, vegetables, whole grains, wild-caught fish high in omega-3 fatty acids (salmon, tuna, etc.), and other anti-inflammation foods.

If you smoke or use other nicotine products, try to quit. Smoking is associated with increased inflammation and pain.

See a video about *How to Make 5 Quick and Easy Ice Packs*:
spine-health.com/ebook/cnp/link6

7.

MEDICAL TREATMENTS

When neck pain is not successfully managed with self-care, or if you have a recurrence of symptoms, it may be necessary to visit a doctor for an evaluation and to explore other medical treatment options.

PRESCRIPTION PAIN-RELIEF MEDICATIONS

Some form of medication may be part of a treatment plan for chronic neck pain, especially for short periods such as during a flare-up.

Using the correct type and amount of medication can be important to managing and recovering from neck pain. For example, completely avoiding medication could allow pain levels to remain high enough to interfere with sleep and the ability to enjoy normal activities, which may cause depression or other mood problems. On the other hand, taking the wrong medication type or dosage could cause serious side effects.

If over-the-counter pain medications, such as acetaminophen or nonsteroidal anti-inflammatories (NSAIDs), are not adequately controlling the pain, your doctor may recommend a prescription medication. Some examples include:

- **PRESCRIPTION-STRENGTH NSAIDS.** These medications target inflammation, which is the source of the pain. Prescription-strength NSAIDs tend to be stronger than over-the-counter NSAIDs, but they may also have higher risks for serious side effects, including heart, kidney, and gastrointestinal. Although, the potential benefits and risks can vary based on your individual health status and the specific medication. For example, some people may experience fewer gastrointestinal side effects from a prescription-strength NSAID called celecoxib (COX-2 inhibitor), but others may not.

- **MUSCLE RELAXANTS.** For unrelenting muscle spasms, a muscle relaxant such as methocarbamol may be prescribed. Muscle relaxants are also only for short-term use because they can have serious side effects. Further, muscle relaxants help with muscle spasms in the short term but they do not help address the underlying reason for the muscle spasm.

- **OPIODS.** Also known as narcotic pain medications, opioids are typically used for severe pain over a relatively short period of time (1 or 2 weeks) when other lower-risk medications have not provided relief. Longer use increases the risk for developing drug dependency, addiction, or other side effects, such as sleepiness, dizziness, nausea, breathing problems, and constipation.

Many other prescription medications are also available for treating neck pain, including drugs that may specifically target nerve pain, such as some anti-seizure medications and antidepressants.

Remember that medication only helps to reduce pain symptoms and does not cure the underlying cause of pain. Think of the medication as part of your broader treatment plan, enabling you to continue with getting better sleep, staying active with walking, and regularly performing neck exercises and stretches.

PHYSICAL THERAPY

An exercise program designed by a physical therapist or other certified medical professional can target muscles in the neck, upper back, and core. Strengthening and stretching these muscles can reduce the risks associated with poor posture, such as muscle spasms, that may worsen your symptoms. See chapter 8 for details about some helpful therapeutic exercises and stretches.

INJECTIONS

Typically one of the last non-surgical treatments to be tried, various injection options are available for the cervical spine, including:

- **CERVICAL FACET INJECTION.** This procedure, aided by fluoroscopy and contrast, involves injecting a steroid and local anesthetic solution into a facet joint that is suspected of causing pain. If the injection offers temporary relief for the duration of the local anesthetic used, the facet joint is considered a probable source of pain.

- **CERVICAL EPIDURAL STEROID INJECTION.** With the aid of fluoroscopy (x-ray guidance) and contrast to visualize the needle's location inside the body, a steroid solution is injected into the spinal canal's outer layer, called the epidural space. This injection is normally used to reduce inflammation from a herniated disc and/or inflamed nerve root.

  Watch our video about Cervical Epidural Steroid Injections: spine-health.com/ebook/cnp/link14

- **MEDIAL BRANCH BLOCK.** This procedure involves injecting a lidocaine solution along the sensory nerve that innervates the facet joint. It is purely a diagnostic injection to confirm or refute the facet joints as the cause of pain. After the injection, which is guided by fluoroscopy and contrast, the patient is given a short pain diary to be kept for the next eight hours. If the pain is alleviated for a few hours (about the same amount of time as lidocaine is effective along the nerve), the facet joint is confirmed as the likely source of pain.

- **RADIOFREQUENCY ABLATION (RFA).** In cases when the pain source has been confirmed, RFA may be considered. Using fluoroscopy, a special needle is placed near the facet joint's sensory nerve to target. Then the needle tip is heated by radiofrequency waves to create a heat lesion on the nerve, preventing pain signals from traveling to the brain. RFA may offer longer-lasting relief (typically 6 to 18 months), but the nerve typically grows back. If the same pain recurs after 12 months or so, the procedure can be repeated.

- **TRIGGER POINT INJECTION.** This type of injection's goal is to reset an irritated muscle bundle (or "turn off" an active trigger point), allowing painful muscle spasms to resolve. Trigger point injections can greatly vary in their contents, such as having saline, lidocaine, steroid, or some combination of these. It should be done without injecting anything into the muscle, but if needed for pain, a very small amount of local anesthetic may be used.

Keep in mind that these injections address the inflammation and/or muscle spasms that can cause neck pain, but they do not address the altered biomechanics that may have initially caused these problems. So while the inflammation and/or muscle spasm is improved and the pain is gone or lessened, it is important to use this window of opportunity to address the biomechanics with things like therapeutic exercises, lifestyle modifications, and ergonomic improvements.

While many people have experienced some neck pain relief from injections, serious complications have been reported in rare cases. Discuss the potential benefits and risks with your doctor before deciding on an injection.

SPINAL CORD STIMULATION

A small device (implanted near the pain source in the cervical spine) sends gentle electrical pulses to the spinal cord to modify or mask the pain signals before they travel to the brain. When successful, spinal cord stimulation can change a chronic pain sensation to become more of a tingling or mild pain that enables a return to normal activities and lifestyle.

Spinal cord stimulation requires a trial period of about one week to see if it adequately relieves pain before the device is permanently implanted. Spinal cord stimulation may be tried as a last resort before surgery, or if you want to avoid surgery or prescription painkillers.

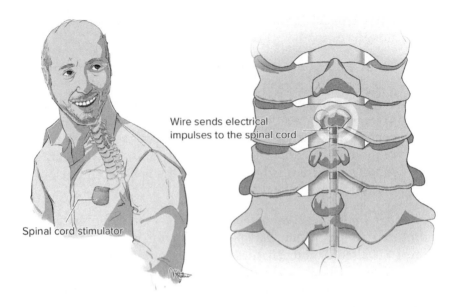

Wire sends electrical impulses to the spinal cord

Spinal cord stimulator

Spinal cord stimulation also has risks associated with implanting the device in the body. It is also possible that the implanted device does not relieve pain as well as the trial did. Spinal cord stimulation is reserved for severe chronic neck pain that has failed to respond to more conservative care.

For more information, read *Treatment for Neck Pain*:
spine-health.com/ebook/cnp/link7

8.

THERAPEUTIC EXERCISES

O ur necks were designed to move, but at least some of that movement is reduced when the neck becomes painful. As such, almost every neck pain treatment plan includes some form of exercise and stretching to help improve the neck's strength and mobility. In addition to boosting mood and potentially reducing pain, exercise can increase blood flow and bring more oxygen and nutrients into the neck.

Before starting any exercise program, it's best to consult with a trained medical professional who is familiar with what you personally can and cannot do. A doctor, physiatrist, physical therapist, or chiropractor can help design an exercise program that starts at an appropriate level for you, then slowly increases the challenge so you can make progress over time. These medical professionals can ensure that you're doing the exercises with proper form, which is crucial for making gains and avoiding injury.

The exercises in this book can be considered a supplement to the program you and your doctor decide is right. Ideally you will discuss these exercises with your doctor and integrate them into your day. Stretches in this book may have different names and modifications. Also, remember to keep breathing throughout every exercise. Sometimes people focus or strain so much on an exercise that they stop breathing, which could increase the risk for serious complications, such as stroke.

STRETCHES

CORNER STRETCH. Standing about 2 feet away, face the corner of a room. With both feet together and elbows slightly beneath shoulder level, place a forearm on each wall. Lean in until you feel a good stretch of the shoulders and chest. Hold the stretch for 30 to 60 seconds. This can be repeated a few times a day.

LEVATOR SCAPULAE STRETCH. While sitting or standing, raise the elbow above the shoulder. With the elbow up, rest it against a door jamb. Then turn the head in the opposite direction and lower the chin, which should stretch the back of the neck on the side that has the elbow raised. To slightly increase the stretch, gently push the back of the head a little further with your fingertips. Hold this stretch for 30 to 60 seconds before switching to the other side. Repeat a few times a day if desired.

POSTERIOR PELVIC TILT WITH CHEST STRETCH. Lie on your back with arms at the side, knees flexed, and feet flat on the ground as if you were about to do a sit-up. Now imagine your belly pushing downward to flatten your stomach until the lower back is also flat against the ground. Slowly bring your arms out to the sides of your body so that you feel a stretch in the front of your chest wall and shoulders. If this is easy, keep bringing them up until you get them directly over your head. Once you feel a stretch, hold this position for 20 seconds. Rest and repeat one time.

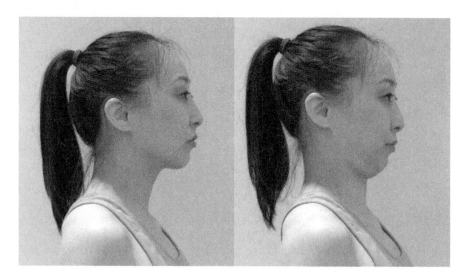

CHIN TUCKS. Starting out, stand with your back against a door jamb and both feet about 3 inches from the bottom of the door. While keeping the spine flat against the door jamb, pull the head straight back until it touches the door jamb. The chin should be kept straight throughout (not looking up). Hold for 5 seconds and repeat 10 times.

Another way to do chin tucks is as follows: While standing or sitting, place your thumb on the sternum and your pinky on the chin. Then keep your hand still while pulling your head straight back (away from the pinky). As you gain experience, you can do chin tucks without the aid of a door jamb or pinky.

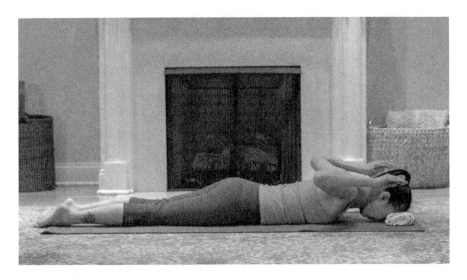

PRONE COBRA. While lying face down on the floor, rest the forehead on a pillow or rolled-up hand towel. Gradually raise your head, chest, and arms upward while keeping the elbows out. Initially, try to raise the forehead at least an inch off the towel. As you get stronger, you can raise the head and chest higher, but the head should always be looking mostly downward to avoid overarching the neck. Squeeze the shoulder blades together and hold the up position for 10 seconds. Repeat 10 times if possible.

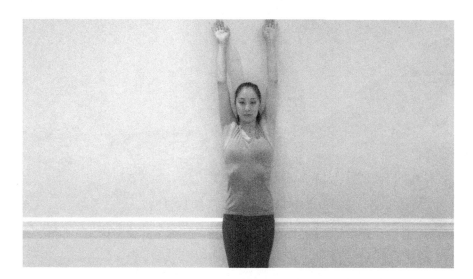

BACK BURN. Stand with the back against the wall and both feet about 4 inches from the bottom of the wall. While keeping the arms and back of hands flat against the wall, raise the hands to about shoulder height and don't let them go lower for the duration of the exercise. Then slowly raise the arms and hands until they're above your head as high as they can go without leaving the wall or causing pain. Then slowly lower them. Repeat 10 times, 3 to 5 times per day.

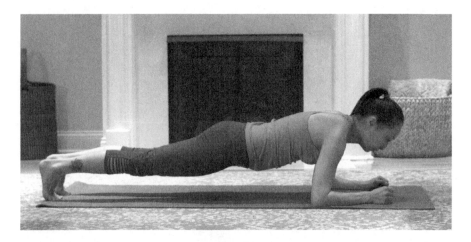

PLANK. Lie flat on a mat and then push up, elevating onto your forearms and toes while keeping the palms and forearms flat on the mat. The torso should be held straight "as a plank." As you hold the position, contract your abdominal muscles and gluteus (buttocks) muscles. Don't allow your buttocks to stick up in the air or sag down. Hold this position for up to one minute but stop as soon as you are unable to remain straight as a plank. As you get stronger over time, try to repeat this exercise three times with 30-second intervals of rest in between.

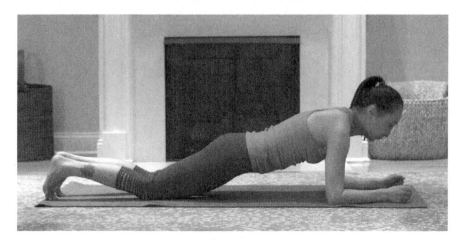

If a regular plank is too difficult, a **MODIFIED PLANK** allows your knees to rest on the ground and then plank upward.

RESISTANCE BAND EXERCISES

Resistance bands are convenient because they're easy to store at home or take on the road. Below are a couple of exercises that target muscles in the back and shoulders, which can help with better posture and reduce neck pain. Start by wrapping the resistance band around a solid anchor that won't move, such as a weight machine at the gym or a metallic door handle that won't slip or break, then:

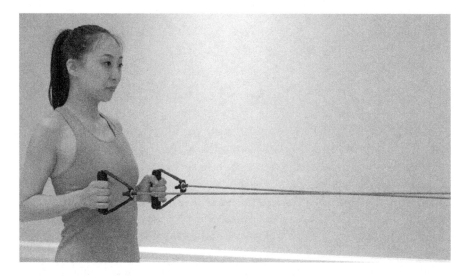

PULL STRAIGHT BACK. Stand with good posture (back straight, ears above the shoulders) and pull the resistance band toward you by flexing the elbows straight back. Inhale slowly while pulling the band back as far as you can, and squeeze your shoulder blades together at the end of the contraction. Hold the shoulder blades together for a count of two and then exhale slowly as you extend your elbows and return to the starting position. Do three sets of 10 repetitions.

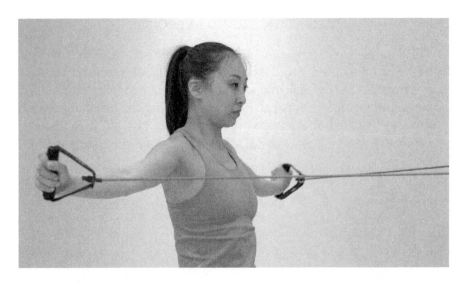

PULL TO THE SIDES. Similar to the previous exercise, stand with good posture but this time keep the arms straight and pull the resistance band toward the sides. Inhale slowly while pulling the band back as far as you can, and squeeze your shoulders at the end of the contraction. Hold the shoulder blades together for a count of two and then exhale slowly as you extend your arms and return to the starting position. Do three sets of 10 repetitions. (If three sets of 10 repetitions becomes relatively easy, choose a heavier resistance band. Also, if you're new to resistance bands, be sure to consult with a physical therapist or other qualified professional before starting.)

For more information, read *Neck Exercises for Neck Pain*:
spine-health.com/ebook/cnp/link8

9.

ALTERNATIVE TREATMENTS

I f neck pain is persistent and not fully relieved by conventional medical treatments, you may want to try alternative or complementary treatments. While alternative treatments may have less or little medical evidence to support their use, many people have reported achieving some neck pain relief by using these methods.

Alternative treatments may be used as a primary approach for managing pain or additional approach to other medical treatment. You may find an alternative treatment to be more tolerable, especially if it can help you reduce the need for pain medications that may have side effects.

MANUAL MANIPULATION

Manual adjustments made to the cervical spine, such as by a chiropractor, osteopath, physical therapist, or other health professional, may help improve range of motion and reduce pain. Manual manipulation is commonly used as part of an overall physical therapy program for neck pain.

There are two general categories for applying an adjustment directly to the neck:

- **CERVICAL SPINE MANIPULATION** is the traditional high-velocity, low-amplitude adjustment commonly associated with chiropractic treatment. This approach involves using the hands to move the neck in a manner that sometimes may cause a minor joint pop or cracking sound. Many times the joint moves without any sound or feeling. Some people find the manipulation helpful and experience relief. Other people may find that high velocity manipulation is psychologically unappealing. Manipulation rarely causes pain during the treatment.

- **CERVICAL SPINE MOBILIZATION** involves using slow but firm movement—either by the hands or a device—to ease the spinal joints through their range of motion. This approach has the same goals as cervical spine manipulation but is less forceful and may be preferred by patients who have certain conditions that could make the neck unstable, such as osteoporosis, or do not like to hear joint cracking (similar to knuckle cracking).

Manual manipulation of the cervical spine is generally a safe procedure. However, there have been extremely rare reports of serious injury during the procedure, such as stroke or injury to the spine. Be sure that your chiropractor or other medical professional is licensed and capable of evaluating whether your cervical spine can safely tolerate manual manipulation.

ACUPUNCTURE

Acupuncture involves placing ultra-thin needles into the body at specific points depending on the pain type and/or location being treated. This therapy is based on the belief that an energy imbalance is causing the pain, and the strategic placement of the needles may help restore the energy balance throughout the body.

Acupuncturists theorize that there are more than 2,000 acupuncture points in the body connected by 20 energy channels called "meridians." For this reason, while the pain may be in your neck, it would not be uncommon for an acupuncturist to place needles in your ear, scalp, leg, and/or feet. Sometimes, depending on the school and style of acupuncture, the acupuncturist may place no needles in your neck.

While science has yet to validate the existence of meridians or the effectiveness of acupuncture, many people have reported that this therapy helped them recover from neck pain or at least achieve some temporary relief.

When performed by a licensed acupuncturist, the procedure is considered relatively safe. However, it is not commonly covered by insurance and could be expensive.

MASSAGE THERAPY

A neck and shoulder massage may help increase blood flow, relax muscles, increase range of motion, and ease stress, among other potential benefits. All of these factors can play a role in helping to reduce neck pain, even if it is just temporary relief. Massage therapy is commonly combined with other treatments, such as heat therapy and/or physical therapy.

While some people may get enough relief by massaging their own neck or having a partner do it, others might experience better results from a professional massage. Various types of massages are available, such as Swedish massage, Shiatsu massage, deep-tissue massage, and others.

MINDFUL PAIN MANAGEMENT

Some studies have shown that practicing mindfulness and meditation may help relax the body and reduce the sensation of pain. There are various forms of this treatment, but most of them involve controlled breathing exercises to start. Here's one example that is good for beginners:

- Go into a quiet room and get into a reclined position, such as in a reclining chair or a couch with pillows to prop yourself up comfortably. Close your eyes or focus on a single point in the room.

- Slowly take a deep breath in through your nose. Focus on having the chest pull the air down into your stomach while counting to 10. Then slowly exhale through pursed lips while again counting to 10.

- Repeat this slow, controlled breathing until you feel yourself relaxing.

Once you've slowed down your breathing and are calm, there are many other techniques that you can try, such as:

- **ALTERED FOCUS.** Concentrate on a part of your body that does not hurt, such as your foot. Now imagine your foot gradually having an altered sensation, such as warming up or getting cold. This focus on an altered sensation in a pain-free body part can take your mind off the area that has been hurting.

- **PAIN MOVEMENT.** Focus on the most painful area, such as in your neck or arm. Now imagine that you are taking control of the pain and slowly moving it to a nearby area. If the pain is in your neck, slowly picture it leaving your neck and moving to your shoulder, then your elbow, and eventually into your hand. If you're able to visualize the pain far from its actual source, try imagining the pain floating into the air and completely leaving your body.

Several other techniques are available. Trying mindful pain management 3 times a week for 30 minutes can be a good goal, but your doctor may recommend more or less, depending on your situation.

It is important to remember that mindful pain management is not intended to eliminate your pain. However, with practice, it may help you reduce the pain and/or feel more control over it.

TRANSCUTANEOUS ELECTRICAL NERVE STIMULATION (TENS)

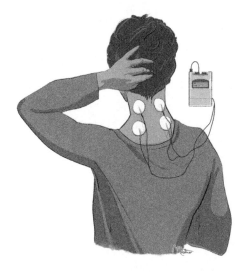

TENS therapy is the most common form of electrotherapy. The theory behind electrotherapy is to send mild electrical pulses to the painful area in an effort to alter sensations and reduce pain.

TENS therapy usually involves a battery-operated unit that sends electrical signals via wires to adhesive electrodes that are attached to the skin. A handheld controller enables you to adjust the current, as well as the stimulation patterns.

For some people, the TENS unit gives them a mild tingling that reduces or masks the pain. However, not everyone experiences benefits and there are some risks, such as the possibility of developing a skin rash. Most patients experiment with a TENS unit for a week or two at physical therapy or a chiropractor's office before committing to buy one for home use.

For more information, read *Transcutaneous Electrical Nerve Stimulators (TENS)*: spine-health.com/ebook/cnp/link9

10.

SURGERY FOR NECK PAIN

Most cases of chronic neck pain do not require surgery. However, if you have not found relief from neck pain after trying several nonsurgical treatments over a period of 3 to 6 months, surgery may become an option.

Before having neck surgery, your surgeon will need to image and diagnose the source of the pain. If the source of pain cannot be identified or is unlikely to be fixed by surgery, it is better to forgo surgery and continue with nonsurgical treatments.

ANTERIOR CERVICAL DISCECTOMY AND FUSION (ACDF)

ACDF surgery is considered the gold standard for patients with pain that stems from the discs in the cervical spine. This procedure has several decades of data to support its safety and effectiveness in treating neck and arm pain caused by a compressed nerve in the neck.

HOW ACDF SURGERY WORKS

The first part of ACDF surgery is the discectomy. It typically involves a 1- or 2-inch incision on the right or left side of the neck. The thin layer of muscle beneath the skin is cut and moved aside, then the remaining soft tissues are dissected until the intervertebral disc is exposed. Using fluoroscopy (x-ray guidance), the surgeon places a needle into the disc space to confirm that the correct vertebral level has been reached. The damaged disc is removed, and other tissues may also be removed, such as nearby ligaments or bone spurs.

After the damaged disc and any other problematic materials are removed, the cervical fusion can be set up. A bone graft is inserted in place of the removed disc in order to maintain normal spacing between the vertebrae and allow enough room for the nerve roots to exit the spinal canal unimpeded. (The bone graft may come from your hip bone, which would require another incision, or from a donor bone or bone graft substitute.) A small metal plate is then placed at the front of the adjacent vertebrae to hold them in place while the fusion starts to heal together.

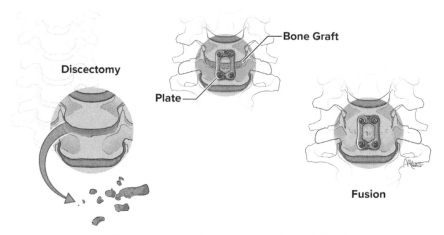

POSTOPERATIVE CARE AFTER ACDF

Modern ACDF surgeries typically enable the patient to go home a few hours after the procedure. In some cases, the patient may need to stay overnight for further observation and care.

During the first week or two of recovery at home, it makes sense to have a family member, friend, or home health aide to help with chores and check on you. Many activities are restricted early on, including:

- **BENDING, LIFTING, AND TWISTING.** Examples include cooking, gardening, doing laundry, caring for young children or pets, or lifting anything heavier than a gallon of milk (about 8 pounds).

- **BATHS AND SHOWERS.** While the incision site's wound is healing, it must stay dry and clean to avoid infection. No baths or any type of submersion in water is allowed. After 2 or 3 days, showers may be allowed if care is taken to prevent the wound from becoming wet.

- **DRIVING.** No driving is allowed while on prescription pain medications that affect alertness and reaction times, such as opioids. Some patients are cleared to drive about 2 weeks after surgery, but others take longer.

- **SOLID FOODS.** While the throat is healing, liquids and soft foods are recommended the first few days. Then solid foods are slowly added back into your diet.

Recovery times from ACDF surgery can vary greatly. Some patients with a sedentary job, such as office work that is done at a desk, may start returning to work 3 or 4 days after surgery if the pain is sufficiently reduced and energy levels are increasing. Other patients may take a full 2 weeks or longer before starting to feel better, at which point a physical rehabilitation program is likely to begin and could take up to 3 months to complete. Returning to more strenuous activities, such as a construction job or contact sports, could take 3 to 6 months, or longer. If more than one level is required to be fused, this will increase the amount of recovery time as well.

See a video about ACDF: spine-health.com/ebook/cnp/link10

PAIN MANAGEMENT

Managing pain is an important part of the ACDF recovery process, especially in the beginning. Once the medication starts to wear off after surgery, the following types of pain are common:

- Pain and swelling at the throat's incision site (and at the hip's incision site if the bone graft was taken from there)

- Muscle tightness or intense spasm in the upper back and shoulders

- Ongoing neck pain, numbness, and/or tingling

- Pain that worsens with activity, such as when getting out of bed or a chair

- Reduced ability to sleep due to pain or soreness

To successfully manage these pain symptoms while recovering from ACDF, one or more of the following treatments may help:

- **PAIN MEDICATIONS.** During the first week or two, you will likely be given prescription pain medications, such as opioids, and then gradually transition to milder medications, such as acetaminophen (Tylenol). Keep in mind that some opioid medications are combined with acetaminophen, so always check with your doctor or pharmacist to ensure that you are not accidentally overdosing on acetaminophen, which can be dangerous.

- **COLD AND/OR HEAT THERAPY.** During the first 24 to 48 hours after your surgery, cold therapy can be especially useful for minimizing inflammation, swelling, and pain. After a couple days, you may apply heat therapy or cold therapy depending on your preferences. See chapter 6 for more details about applying cold or heat therapy.

- **WALKING.** One of the best things you can do after ACDF surgery is to take short walks. It improves blood circulation, which helps bring more oxygen and nutrients throughout the body, including the tissues that are healing. Walking also can help boost your mood, reduce pain, and lower the risk for developing severe constipation, which can be a problem for some people on opioids after surgery.

- **SLEEP SUPPORT.** You may find it difficult to sleep due to pain and discomfort during the early days of your recovery. Whatever position you find to be most comfortable to fall asleep tends to be recommended, except for sleeping on your stomach, which puts the most stress on the cervical spine. In the days following an ACDF, most people find that sleeping in a reclined position is best. Try using extra pillows to prop yourself up in bed, or sleep in a reclining chair.

Many other methods for managing pain during your ACDF recovery period exist, such as mindful pain management (mentioned in chapter 9).

POSTOPERATIVE REHABILITATION

Most ACDF patients are recommended to start a physical therapy program about 4 weeks after surgery. By this time you should be feeling better and have improved energy levels, but the physical therapy is still important for strengthening and stretching the neck for better range of motion and to reduce the risk of pain returning.

Specific rehabilitation recommendations for ACDF patients can vary widely, depending on different medical opinions and the needs of the specific patient. However, most physical therapy programs for ACDF patients start with basic stretching and gradually work in more exercises over an 8-week period. See chapter 8 for therapeutic exercises you can also do on your own after consulting and reviewing them with your surgeon.

RISKS ASSOCIATED WITH ACDF SURGERY

ACDF surgery is a relatively safe and effective procedure when performed on a good candidate by a well-trained surgeon. However, every surgery has risks for serious complications, such as infection or excessive bleeding. Some other risks associated with ACDF include:

- **FAILURE TO FUSE.** Also called pseudarthrosis, it is possible for the bone graft to not fuse. This problem can result in chronic inflammation and pain remaining in the area where the vertebral bones are failing to grow together and heal.

- **REDUCED ABILITY TO SWALLOW AND/OR SPEAK.** An ACDF surgery is done in close proximity to the esophagus and other soft tissues of the neck, so this area typically experiences inflammation and swelling. It is common for patients to have some difficulty with speaking and/or swallowing for a couple days or weeks following the procedure, but in rare cases these abilities are permanently reduced or lost.

- **NERVE ROOT DAMAGE.** If a nerve root is damaged during the procedure, continued pain, numbness, weakness, and/or paralysis may occur in the arm.

- **DURAL TEAR.** If the outer layer of the spinal cord (dura mater) gets nicked, it can result in a cerebrospinal fluid leak that may cause severe headaches and other symptoms.

- **SPINAL CORD DAMAGE.** While extremely rare, an injury to the spinal cord during the procedure can have serious consequences, such as loss of a bodily function or paralysis in one or more limbs.

- **ADJACENT SEGMENT DISEASE.** After ACDF, the mechanical forces that used to go through the now-fused spinal segment get shifted to the adjacent unfused (still mobile) segments above and below the fusion. This in turn creates increased pressure on those cervical spine levels and may lead to increased wear-and-tear, potentially causing problems as time marches on.

Other complications may also occur, and risk can be affected by your unique health history. Before opting for ACDF surgery, ask your surgeon about the procedure's overall risks and if your case requires any special considerations.

ARTIFICIAL DISC REPLACEMENT SURGERY

A newer but still established procedure, cervical artificial disc replacement (ADR), removes the problematic disc in the same manner as ACDF. However, instead of inserting a bone graft to set up a solid fusion, an artificial disc is implanted to maintain motion between the vertebrae.

Long-term data on cervical ADR is still being gathered, so its effectiveness and risks are not yet as well-studied as ACDF. Of the research collected thus far, results have been promising for cervical ADR's efficacy to be comparable to ACDF while maintaining more of the cervical spine's natural motions and not leading to as much increased stress on adjacent levels.

OTHER SURGICAL OPTIONS

Depending on where the problematic degeneration is located in your cervical spine, other surgical options may be available or done in addition to the procedures previously mentioned. These procedures may include:

- **CERVICAL LAMINECTOMY.** This surgery involves the removal of the lamina, which is the vertebra's bony arch that protects the back of the spinal cord. In some cases, enough spinal decompression is achieved to relieve symptoms by removing the lamina alone. Sometimes a laminectomy can be done without a fusion. A similar procedure, called a laminoplasty, involves restructuring the lamina to create more room, rather than completely removing it.

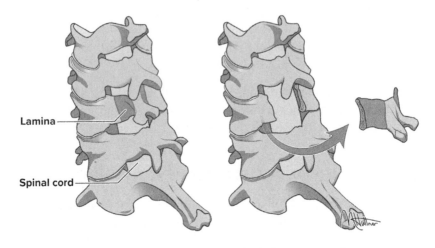

Removal of the spinous process and laminae (shaded) in a cervical laminectomy surgery.

- **CERVICAL FORAMINOTOMY.** A small part of the foramen (bony opening where the nerve root exits the spinal canal) is removed. This procedure may just remove a problematic bone spur, or it could be more extensive with the partial removal of a disc and/or other soft tissues that were compressing the nerve root in the foramen. This procedure may be done with or without a fusion.

- **CERVICAL CORPECTOMY.** Rarely performed, this surgery is much more extensive than the other procedures mentioned in this chapter as it involves the complete removal of a vertebral body, as well as the adjacent discs above and below. A corpectomy is typically employed when spinal stenosis is causing spinal cord compression at multiple levels.

Surgery for neck pain is commonly done at one or sometimes two vertebral levels, but occasionally it is needed at more levels. The more levels involved in the surgery, the greater the potential risk for complications, including the risk of subsequent adjacent segment disease.

For more information, read *Surgery for Neck Pain Symptoms*: spine-health.com/ebook/cnp/link11

11.

WRAP-UP

Neck pain that lasts for weeks or months can be disheartening, but don't lose hope. Many treatments are available, and most people eventually find relief after experimenting with different combinations of treatments.

Hopefully, this book has given you a better understanding of what may be causing your neck pain, as well as some treatment ideas to try. Be persistent and patient as you apply different treatments, carefully following directions and giving them ample time to work. In rare cases when 3 to 6 months of nonsurgical treatments don't provide enough neck pain relief to resume normal activity levels, a surgical consultation may be considered.

Living an overall healthy lifestyle is a good way to naturally take care of your body and minimize the risk for developing neck pain. Staying active, exercising, stretching, using good posture, eating healthy, not smoking, and getting the recommended amounts of sleep every night are all smart moves to keep your neck at its best.

For more information on this topic and a full range of other spinal conditions, including educational videos, detailed articles, discussion forums, and interviews with spine specialists, visit Spine-health.com, your source for accurate, unbiased information and treatment options.

For more information on neck pain symptoms, visit our Neck Pain Health Center: spine-health.com/ebook/cnp/link12

THANK YOU FOR READING!

For more information and additional resources on chronic neck pain, visit us on the web at **Spine-health.com.**

Printed in Great Britain
by Amazon

27852671R00036